"*Although the book is short and very easy to read, it packs powerful information for all readers to understand what is headache, what causes it, and how is it treated, no matter what the reader's background is. As a dentist myself, I found the description of the anatomy and physiology simple but accurate, which is challenging to do as the human body is so wonderfully complex. I applaud the author on his excellent job in doing this, and I will be stealing some of the ways he explain things to use for my patients.*"
    –Kevin L

Please don't forget to visit Amazon.com and leave a review! Thank you!

See what people are saying about
Hidden Secrets of Migraine Headaches on
Amazon.com!

"This book is a well-organized orientation for migraine sufferers with some insights as to why headaches occur and where to turn for help. In particular, the author points out the fact that some patients should look to their dentist for solutions and not only their physician. If you are someone who suffers from severe headaches and have not talked to a dentist, this little book may be very useful in helping you identify alternative causes as well as new treatment options that you have not yet pursued or considered."
 -Joy Nelson

"Knock on wood, I have never experienced a migraine. That being said, both my daughter and wife have!...who could have imagined that a dental surgeon was the answer. My dear ones have suffered from headaches for the past few months and this provides another opportunity and possible answer - I will pass the soft cover along as soon as available - thank you Dr. Wang, for providing this important insight!"
 -Bruce Langevin

"Well-written, concise, and informative. I learned a lot from this book regarding migraines and a lot of the information provided in the book will be helpful to those who are suffering or know someone suffering from migraines. Easily recommended!"
    –Joey Y

"The book gives much more than I was expecting. The author is clearly a specialist in this subject and there is plenty of technical information given. This would valuable reading for both medical and dental practitioners as well as head pain sufferers. Readers are given a clear direction as to the type of healthcare provider to assess and treat head pain, and the methods used. The results? 'When properly assessed, our treatment success-rate is greater than 93% in reducing the intensity, frequency and duration of chronic pain'."
    –Stephen Parr

Hidden Secrets of Migraine Headaches

5 Keys Dentists Possess in Providing You Lasting Migraine and Other Chronic Pain Relief

Dr. Cheng Lun Wang

Table of Contents

Introduction

Whenever you see dentists portrayed in movies or on television, you will see the dentist holding a drill or a big needle full of Novocain. It is a given that dentists deal with pain every day and must learn ways to control them effectively.

The first time I used a needle on a real person was during the beginning of our clinical term in third-year dental school. All of the third-year dental students gathered in the main clinic—you could see the tension in everyone's eyes and even in some people's hands as we prepared to perform our very first injection, using each other as guinea pigs. The idea was to pair up, and we would try to do a nerve-block on each other. We had learned all the anatomy and physiology and pharmacology about this procedure, but now we had to actually do it. It was a relatively easy procedure that, as practicing dentists, we would do every day. On that day, I injected my partner with Lidocaine, which is supposed to freeze the nerve in question for about 2 hours. Well, I hit the jackpot that day—I actually nicked the major nerve to the lower jaw with my needle, which is rarely done, and when that happens, the freezing can be very profound. In this case, the freezing lasted around 8 hours!

Over the next two years, we learned all about drilling and filling and other fun dental stuff. But most of all, we learned about pain control in the head and neck areas, which is crucial before, during and after most procedures. There is another type of pain that we deal with on a daily basis that is persistent: chronic pain.

According to the World Health Organization, 1 in 20 people in the developed world suffer with a daily tension headache. 150 million workdays are lost annually to headaches. Over 12% of North Americans suffer from migraine every year. Has chronic head-pain reached epidemic proportions? With all our advances in modern medicine, why have we not found a cure for headaches? Yes, there are all kinds of treatments for headaches, and millions of patients benefit from it; however, there is a large group of chronic head-pain patients who have eluded all conventional medical treatments.

Chronic headaches and migraines are typically treated by physicians, which is the right place to start in most cases. However, over 80% of pain conditions in the head and neck areas actually involve the oral cavity and the jaw. Injuries resulting from improper force on the muscles, joints and other soft tissues in the oral cavity and in the head and neck areas contribute to a large percentage of chronic headaches and migraines. These patients with a complex set of symptoms including tinnitus, vertigo, and others, collectively describe a condition called Dentomandibular Sensorimotor Dysfunction (DMSD).

Until recently, there has not been a way to properly and systematically assess this condition, leading to partial or ineffective treatment. The breakthrough came with the realization that we must incorporate the expertise of advanced dentistry and medical rehabilitation techniques in order to address the needs of this type of head-pain. A combination of technologically advanced assessment tools from both medicine and dentistry is used to pinpoint areas of injury. Dentists, with their basic medical training and extensive knowledge in the head and neck areas, are the best choice to carry out these assessments and procedures.

In this book, we will talk about the hidden secrets that have kept so many chronic head-pain patients from finding effective, lasting relief from their pain. We will examine why they have tried every type of treatment out there and are still suffering. We will discuss the frequent causes of chronic pain in the head and neck areas, and all the symptoms associated with these disorders. Best of all, we will talk about effective treatment for chronic headache sufferers. I will explain why these cases have slipped through the cracks of our medical system, and why dentists hold the key for solving them. Since 1 in 5 people in the general public will have suffered one or more of these pain conditions in the past year, the assessment and treatment we talk about here will be essential to you or someone you know.

Chapter 1

My Personal Journey.

If someone told me that I would be diagnosing and treating patients with chronic head-pain on the day that I entered dental school 31 years ago, I would have thought *they* were the ones with chronic head problems. At the time, my knowledge of what a dentist does, similar to what the general public still believes, was that they poked around in people's mouths, finding rotten teeth and fixing them. As we went through the first two years of dental school, we took courses in anatomy, physiology, pathology and pharmacology, all with medical students. Back then, I believed that the study of these general medical courses was only useful in helping me in understanding their application in dentistry; however, as I learned more throughout my career, I have come to understand that the fundamentals we learned in dental school served me well in my pursuit in connecting dentistry with medicine and other healthcare techniques.

My four years in dental school at the University of Western Ontario culminated in 1989, with the addition of "Doctor of Dental Surgery" accompanying my name. I went on to an internship at the Hospital for Sick Children in Toronto, followed by a year as resident dentist at the IWK Health Centre in Halifax. The experience working with children helped me with my ultimate decision to become an orthodontist. The privilege of working with someone in a positive environment over an extended period of time, producing pleasing and confident smiles—that is often a life-changing experience, and was exactly what I was looking for as a career.

I entered the graduate orthodontic program at the University of Manitoba in 1991, wanting to learn all there was to learn in the world of orthodontics. I enjoyed learning all the different techniques and innovations, and especially all the gadgets that come with new technologies. At that time, bonding techniques had advanced far enough that gluing braces to teeth was a standard procedure. Patients no longer had to endure silver bands that covered the whole tooth, that famous "train tracks" look, just to have the braces on their teeth. Braces became smaller and smaller as the glue got better and better. Clear braces were invented, and even "invisible" lingual braces (braces glued to the backs of the teeth) became available.

In 1994, I graduated from the orthodontic program with a certificate of orthodontic specialty and a Master of Science degree. I took all my knowledge to Vancouver, Canada, to begin my career as a "tooth straightener" in private practice. At the same time, I wanted to give back to the educational system that gave me my skills, by teaching in the Faculty of Dentistry at the University of British Columbia. I knew then that the best way to keep a curious mind is to be surrounded by people with the same pursuit. Young men and women who are thinking, learning and asking questions are the ones that challenge you to do the same. This has never been truer as I gain more experience and years in private practice. When we work in the same place year after year, it is easy to get into a routine, getting better at what we do; but it is also easy to stop looking for new methods, different solutions, to innovate. Learning institutions and professional meetings tend to encourage this. Being in private practice allowed me to convert those theoretical innovations into practical solutions, which in turn allowed me to create better results.

One day while at work about three years ago, I had a young man come in for a consultation. Dennis is in his late teens, and had finished his orthodontic treatment years before. I was happy to see him; it is always nice to see our patients transform from awkward teenagers into young men and women. It is a pleasure to hear about their pursuits in life, and exciting new challenges they are now facing. However, in this particular case, his experience had not been as encouraging; before me sat a sullen, quiet young man with dim eyes. He was accompanied by his mother, who appeared to be discouraged and agitated. He spoke very little, and we got the story mainly from his mother.

According to Mom, it appears that Dennis has a problem with his bite. Although he had braces years ago with a very good result, a recent car accident has caused his bite to shift. After hearing this, I had Dennis sit down in my examination chair, tipped him back and had a look at his teeth. What I saw surprised me: his teeth were still fairly straight, but his lower jaw was shifted way to the left, such that when he bit down, his upper and lower teeth met way off center, way off balance, in an awkward position.

Having been in private practice for almost twenty years at that time, I had completed thousands of orthodontic cases, and had followed some of them for over fifteen years. I had rarely seen a change in a person's bite of this magnitude. Natural changes after orthodontic treatment are common; they usually come in two forms: teeth may want to shift back toward their original crooked position, which we call orthodontic relapse, or there can be some changes in jaw position due to growth. Now, Dennis was in his late teens, so he undoubtedly experienced some growth changes in the past five years. However, the amount and type of changes I saw seemed impossible; such growth change is something that I should have noticed earlier, during the few years of his orthodontic treatment.

I now turned my attention to the nature and extent of his car accident. Going over the history and treatment of his injuries, it was revealed that he was knocked unconscious on the day of the accident, but was not treated for broken bones in his face or jaw. A CT scan was done at the hospital, and broken bones and other damages were not diagnosed. My questioning did reveal that since he accident, Dennis had had pain in his neck and back every day, with headaches 2-3 times a week as an extension of the neck pain. In fact, since his initial treatment and release from the hospital, Dennis had been treated with physiotherapy and a series of medication, all with no real success. Some of the medications caused significant side effects that made his life miserable, so he soon stopped all forms of prescription medication. The strain of the constant headaches rendered him unable to work or study. The pain and hopelessness of the situation quickly lead to clinical depression. Luckily, Dennis's parents were there to help; they moved him into the basement of their home, where there was less noise and bright lights, which can aggravate his headaches. They sought out alternative treatment for their son, and now settled on medical marijuana daily to help control the pain and depression. They realized this was an untenable situation for a young man with hope for a happy, productive life, and the weight of their circumstance caused a considerable strain on the whole family.

As you can image, with the seriousness of the headache situation, Dennis's dental problems took a back seat. Now, with Dennis's headache situation at a standstill, his mother was still concerned with his overall wellbeing; thus she made the appointment with me to see if there was anything we could do about his teeth. I realized that the source of Dennis's head-pain, depression and jaw and teeth misalignment most likely originated with the car accident injuries; however, at that time I felt that, while I could certainly help him with the jaw problems, I couldn't possibly do anything for his headaches.

At that point in my career, I had not started my BC Head-Pain Institute. I had not made the connection and the subsequent training needed to assess and treat these conditions. Like most dentists and dental specialists, I had concentrated my efforts in honing my skills at treating conditions involving the teeth and the jaw.

Have you ever noticed that, as in most fields of practice, we concentrate on doing what we do best, and we tend to ignore the rest? There is a famous quote by Donald Rumsfeld, State Secretary of Defense in 2002: "As we know, there are known knowns; there are things we know we know. We also know there are known unknowns; that is to say we know there are some things we do not know. But there are also unknown unknowns—the ones we don't know we don't know. And if one looks throughout the history of our country and other free countries, it is the latter category that tend to be the difficult ones." In the case a young man comes to see me for crooked teeth and jaw, as well as headaches, as a dentist I will readily jump in with the crooked teeth, and ignore the rest, because I just didn't know anything about headaches being connected to his crooked jaw.

Something about this situation piqued my interest in headaches, however—probably because it was an unusually desperate situation that happened to my own patient that I had treated for braces over a long period of time, and perhaps because it was a young man that was just coming up to the prime of his life with no real future. This case continued to percolate in the back of my brain as I continued on with my orthodontic practice of happy patients. A couple of months passed by, until one day, I happened upon a small sales booth at a dental meeting that changed my situation from "not knowing what I do not know" to one of "knowing what I do not know." A little glimmer of light appeared in my field of vision to the head-pain world.

Chapter 2

Who Suffers from Chronic Migraines and Headaches?

"... head-pain is one of the top causes for doctor visits. Even with those numbers, surveys suggest that up to 80% of headache sufferers actually do not seek medical help."

1. According to the World Health Organization, 1 in 20 people in the developed world suffer with a daily tension headache.

2. 35 million people in the United States experience migraines every year.

3. 2% of the population have chronic migraine with only 20% of these individuals having received formal diagnosis.

4. Chronic headaches are defined as having 15 or more headaches a month for more than 3 months.

5. 16% of those people who visits the dentist are doing so because of some kind of pain in the mouth, face or head.

There I was, standing in front of this small booth during a coffee break, at a dental convention in California; I see a sign that says "Life-Changing Dentistry." Curious as to what this could be referring to, I asked the salesman there what he was selling. He told me this company created a system for diagnosing and treating patients with headaches and migraines. While going through how this could be used in my practice, he listed off the signs and symptoms of a typical patient that we could treat. As he spoke, the hair on the back of my neck stood up. I began to realize that he was describing *all* of the symptoms my patient Dennis had, and more!

I spent the next hour standing in front of the booth, demanding more answers. By the end of the hour I had a new view of the relationship between headaches and dentistry. Over the next year, I took numerous courses on headaches from a dental perspective, started to look at the scientific literature on headaches and migraine, refreshed myself on all the past learning I had done during my years of dental education, examining it from a new, broader angle, to see how all the pieces fit together. It's like finding a whole new dimension in our existing world!

I can tell you that there is a lot of science behind the connection of head-pain to our dental training; however, we have been too focused on what is going on inside the mouth. Apparently, the same thing applies to the medical field. There is a lot of scientific research done on head-pain. Practically speaking, however, treatment for these head-pain patients has been segregated by the two professions, medical and dental. Out in the real world, diagnosis and treatment of these patients are done only by either the medical professionals or dental professionals. I now realize that we have to treat the patient from both perspectives at the same time in order to be successful with some of the more complex cases.

In short, after I made the connection between headache treatment and the dental profession, I looked forward to being able to help solve Dennis's problems. In addition, once I know what I am looking for in this type of patient, I began to see the problem in many of my own past patients. I guess it's like when you buy a new car which is not a common car— you never noticed them on the road before, but after driving around in it for a week, you notice them all over the place. Since the problem with head-pain in relation to dentistry came onto my radar, I am seeing them everywhere.

Is chronic headache really that big of a problem? Just to give you some background, over 35 million chronic headache-pain sufferers are reported each year in the United States. According to the American Academy of Pain Medicine, 150 million workdays are lost annually to headaches. In Canada, about 30% of Canadians suffered more than one headache per month. Another report found in the *Journal of the American Dental Association* (JADA, October 2015) declares that more than 16% of the North Western US public that visited a dentist in 2014 suffered from orofacial pain—pain originating from teeth, jaw and face—and half of those people suffer from pain of muscle, soft tissues and jaw joint. When you consider these numbers together, it would suggest that about 1 in 5 suffer from pain in the head and neck regions this year alone. Imagine what that means: 1 in 5 people you know suffer from chronic head-pain. If you are a student, about 7 people in your classroom are sufferers; if you are a bus driver, there are 10 sufferers on your bus during rush hour; 4 sufferers in your yoga class; a fifth of the people in your work place, and 100 of your Facebook friends (if you're popular) ... on and on. It would also mean one person in your immediate family is suffering right now!

In fact, head-pain is one of the top causes for doctor visits. Even with those numbers, surveys suggest that up to 80% of headache sufferers actually do not seek medical help. It is no wander that numerous published articles suggest that headaches have reached epidemic proportions.

To be able to treat all these patients, we must first be able define headaches and their causes. Here is where it is going to get a little technical, and I may lose some of you to the details and medical terms. But for those of you willing to stick with me, or in fact enjoy knowing some medical tidbits, this will be very interesting and educational, as we go through some of the anatomy and physiology behind what causes pain, how it is perceived and processed by your brain and thus how it becomes chronic and hard to diagnose.

Chapter 3

What is a Headache, Anyway?

"Pain is an unpleasant sensory and emotional experience associated with actual or potential tissue damage, or described in terms of such damage."

"... headache is not an actual single disorder, but is a symptom that can occur in different conditions."

W hat is a headache? This may seem like a redundant question; you might say, "It is obviously pain in my head!" *Head*, in fact, includes structures such as the jaw, ears, eyes and so on, and we would say that we have an earache if it was localized in the ear. For me, as a dentist, I see toothaches all the time. However, some of the time the toothache is not so obvious; it may actually be a sinus infection, and not from the tooth itself. We cannot actually point to a specific structure and say "This is where all the headaches occur." So actually pinpointing the location of a headache can be difficult and the term becomes ill-defined. At times a "headache" can include many anatomical structures, such as the neck, the ear, the jaw and so on. The Mayo

Clinic defines headaches as "pain in any region of the head. Headaches may occur on one or both sides of the head, be isolated to a certain location, radiate across the head from one point, or have a viselike quality. A headache may appear as a sharp pain, a throbbing sensation or a dull ache."

Next we need to explore the word "ache." We generally assume it to be pain. So let's look at the definition of pain. Merriam-Webster defines pain as "the physical feeling caused by disease, injury, or something that hurts the body". It goes on to define pain as "mental or emotional suffering: sadness caused by some emotional or mental problem". Because it is a complex, subjective phenomenon, that includes physical and psychological components, defining pain has been a challenge. The International Association for the Study of Pain's widely used definition states: "Pain is an unpleasant sensory and emotional experience associated with actual or potential tissue damage, or described in terms of such damage." In medical diagnosis, pain is a symptom. In fact, the International Association for the Study of Pain holds regular conferences where the definition of pain is argued, discussed and updated.

Therefore, *headache* is not an actual single disorder, but is a symptom that can occur in different conditions. For the sake of our discussion here, we will need to include *headache* as one part of the symptoms discussed in the pain of head and face.

We generally divide headaches into different sub groups. First, they can be divided into *acute* or *chronic*. An acute headache is pain or discomfort that starts suddenly and gets worse quickly. Without prior history, this type of headache usually has a physical cause, such as a brain aneurysm, carbon monoxide poisoning or physical trauma.

Chronic daily headaches are defined by the International Headache Society as a headache disorder whereby patients suffer 15 or more headache attacks per month for 3 or more months. Again, you can see it is an arbitrary set of circumstance that defines a condition without specific causes.

Migraine is often used when people describe the worst kind of headaches. Clinically, migraines are actually a different group of head-pain that have certain features. These features may include:

1. Sensitivity to lights or sounds

2. Only occur on one side of the head
3. Visual "aura" such as bright lights and blobs, zigzag lines or distortions in the size or shape of objects before the attack
4. Nausea

There are different kinds of migraines, based on their symptoms, but migraines are usually neurovascular in nature.

All chronic headaches can be classified as *primary* or *secondary*. Primary headaches are ones that can not be attributed to another condition, and are divided into types by underlying conditions such as:

1. Tension: muscle contraction
2. Traction: direct irritation of pain-sensitive structures inside or outside of the skull,
3. Inflammatory: body's response to injury or infection, in which inflammatory cells are produced that specifically cause pain response to alert the body that there is a problem
4. Vascular: dilation or constriction of blood vessels in the head

Secondary headaches are one of the symptoms of another condition such as:

1. Medication overuse
2. Extremely high or low blood sugar levels found in diabetics
3. Low oxygen levels in our system from snoring/sleep apnea
4. Depression/stress
5. Caffeine, and its withdrawal

Secondary headaches are due to an underlying structural or chemical problem in the head or neck. This is a very broad group of medical conditions ranging from dental pain or infected teeth or pain from an infected sinus, to life-threatening conditions like bleeding in the brain or infections like encephalitis or meningitis.

This group of headaches also includes those headaches associated with substance abuse and excess use of medications used to treat headaches, a group we call rebound headaches.

Secondary headaches are in fact what cause the majority of complex chronic headaches, because they can be from a variety of sources that are structurally close to each other. The pain pattern is ill-defined; sometimes they only cause pain when they are acting in conjunction with other factors. We will discuss this further in the next two chapters. Traumatic headaches fall into this category and include post-concussion headaches.

Furthermore, headaches can be exacerbated or triggered by:

1. Hormonal changes
2. Lights and sounds
3. Stress
4. Grinding and clenching of your jaw
5. Lack of sleep
6. Over-exertion or fatigue
7. Food sensitivity
8. Others

You may be very confused with all these medical terms and classifications right about now, and it seems like we are further from actually understanding headaches, let alone solving them! And you are right. What I do want you to understand is that:

1. *Headache* is just a term to describe pain that occurs in the face and head region.
2. There are many causes and conditions that can produce headaches.

3. Our understanding of headaches, and therefore the treatment of them, is constantly evolving.

4. Many areas of expertise will be required to reduce or eliminate some of the more complex head-pain conditions.

Chapter 4

Which Parts of the Body Are Involved? An Anatomy and Physiology Lesson.

"To understand where pain comes from, we must first understand each of these systems, what their function is and what their normal state looks like. Then we can start to see what happens when they are injured and how being out of balance can cause pain."

Before we can talk about why we get headaches, we need to get to know a little about the anatomy of head and neck structures.

1. Muscles: providing the force for movement
2. Bones: frame work for a functional structure
3. Ligaments and tendons: connecting muscles to bones and bones to bones
4. Joints: directing the movements
5. Nerves: providing instructions to the muscles by the brain (afferent), and receiving feedback in way of feel and pain to the brain (efferent) through electrical impulses

6. Teeth: to chew
7. Blood circulation: to feed all the above systems, and to give instructions to these systems through chemical means

The anatomy in our head and neck region is made up of these units; the purpose, of course, is to allow us to do stuff like eat. Pain is an integral part of this functional system as a protective mechanism, so that we don't hurt ourselves when we do things required for basic survival. Pain tells us when there is something wrong, such as when we suffer a cut, or when there is a fire burning us. It also tells us when we have overused a muscle, suffered trauma to the bone or joint or when there is something wrong with any of our systems. So when there is a tear in the muscles or soft tissue, or too much pressure in the joint, or a growth or a pinch in the nerve, and so on, we can say that the system is out of balance.

HEALING THERAPY

GOAL IS TO INCREASE HEALING AND REDUCE INJURY

Humans are born with the ability to heal—that is, when we suffer an injury we are able to self-repair. When the system returns to balance again, pain will go away. Sometimes the source of the injury is too great for our body to overcome, and we cannot heal properly; therefore we remain out of balance. This is when we go into chronic pain condition, or we eventually die. Our medical care is based on this fact; we as doctors merely help remove or lessen the source of injury, or we try to speed up the healing, thus tipping the scale toward health, and restoring balance.

To understand where pain comes from, we must first understand each of these systems, what their function is and what their normal state looks like. Then we can start to see what happens when they are injured and how being out of balance can cause pain.

Muscles of the head and neck: Muscles are there to provide force. Contraction or relaxation of a muscle produces force, which is the basis for movement. Therefore, muscles are the engine for movement. What are the primary functions of the muscles in the head and neck areas? There are two primary functions:

1. To move the head so we see around us (the neck muscles)
2. To move the jaw so we can eat, speak and breath (muscles of mastication)

Bones: Bones in general make up the framework of our body, giving us shape, and provide protection to important organs. The bones in the head and neck areas are there to provide protection to the brain and structural support for our eyes, ears, mouth. Bones also provide the framework that allows the head to stay held upright at the top of our body.

Joints: These are articulating surfaces of bones—that is, where movement between bones can occur. Since bones are hard, they cannot rub together, or they will wear out very fast. So joints are made up of cartilage and soft tissue. The soft tissues connect the cartilage to the bone, bone to bone (ligaments), and muscles to bone and cartilage (tendons). The joints are hinges that connect bone to bone, allowing movement of the bones. It also directs and limits the movements, provides cushioning, and is all held together in a neat little capsule. The joints found in the head and neck area are the neck joints, or the cervical spine, and the temporomandibular joint (TMJ). The neck joints allow our head to swivel and the TMJ allows us to speak and chew. Obviously, these are very important functions, so we will delve into them in more detail later.

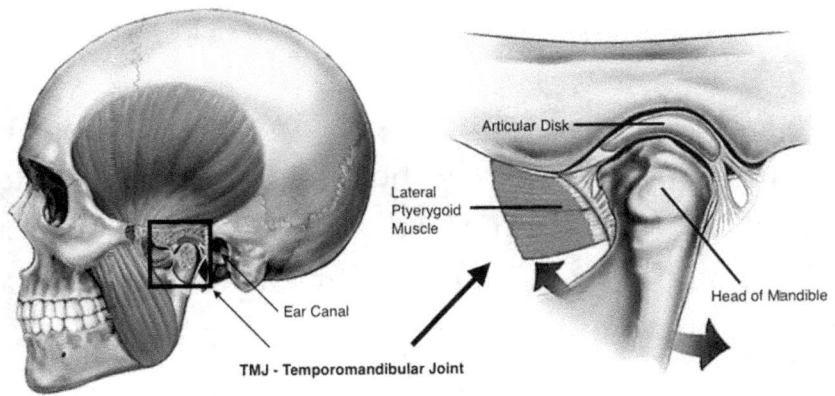

Teeth: We all know what teeth are for: chewing primarily, but they also help in our speech. The masticatory (chewing) system seems to be so simple— just some teeth that come together—but it is actually very complex. In fact, it is of such complexity that it warrants a whole different field of study in our health care system: dentistry.

Nerves: They provide information about various parts of the body to the brain and in turn allow the brain to give instructions to the systems away from the brain. The brain, in fact, is central to this system. The nervous system is the information highway of the body; it runs on electrical impulses and consists of a vast and complex network. It is precisely the complexity of this network which makes it so difficult to diagnose pain. The main nerve that supplies signals for the face, neck, jaw, sinus and teeth is the trigeminal nerve.

Circulatory system: This system provides nutrition to the different parts of the body, and removes wastes and toxins from them as well. It also carries chemical information to and from the different systems, such as hormones and other mediators.

Now that we have a basic understanding of the structures of head and neck, we can begin to talk about what can go wrong to cause pain in this area.

Chapter 5

Why Do We Get Headaches?

"... Therefore, the majority of head-pains, whether it is primary or secondary in nature, are the direct result of pain transmitted, altered, or modified through the trigeminal nucleus."

As described in the last chapter, our body is made up of several systems. These systems all function with particular purpose and have nerves connected to them. Pain in any of these systems is caused by two primary means:

1. Tissue injury pain
2. Nervous system dysfunction pain

Injuries to these systems can be caused by one of the following means:

1. Trauma: specifically, damage to the tissues by excessive force applied to said tissues. Trauma can be divided into macrotrauma, which is a one-time overloading of the tissues by excessive force such as a car accident or sports injury; or

microtrauma, which is the repeated overloading of the tissue over time, eventually resulting in injury, such as nighttime grinding of teeth (known as "bruxing") or runner's shin splints.

2. Infection: a disease process that occurs in the tissues via bacteria or virus that produces injury, such as an abscess or cavity in a tooth.

3. Neoplasm: abnormal growth of certain cells such as cancer cells.

4. Genetic/congenital: abnormal formation or growth of a group of tissues; the way the tissues were programmed to grow is not normal, causing a defect in their formation.

Tissue injuries: These are relatively easy to understand. An injury directly to any tissue, such as muscle or bone or ligament, will usually cause pain because these tissues have nerves connected to them. The injury causes pain signals to be carried to the brain, where the brain interprets the information and recognizes it as pain. Of course, this is a very common phenomenon that occurs to us every day; however, there are situations where our perception of the tissue injury can confuse us—even trained professionals—due to the way our nervous system is wired.

Nervous system dysfunction injuries: This is a type of pain that occurs spontaneously, when there is no pain stimulus in the area where pain is felt. To be more precise, it is a situation where we feel pain in the skin of our cheek when there is nothing wrong with the skin itself. We feel the pain because there is something wrong with the nerves conducting the pain from that region, or there is something wrong with the way our brain interprets signals from that region. This type of pain is caused by a dysfunction of the nerves or brain, and not because of injury to the system itself. One of the most common problems of this type of pain in the face and head area is trigeminal neuralgia (this will be discuss in more detail later), yet even this condition is relatively rare at less than 0.1%.

Referred pain, also known as reflective pain, is a condition where the pain experienced is in a different location from the site of the actual injury. To understand how the signals from one particular part of the body can be misinterpreted by the brain, we have to first understand how our peripheral nervous system is wired. The nerves that are embedded in the different tissues in our body are like fine mesh works. The many wires from one region of the body will come together to one terminal before going to the brain. So the signals from different small wires in one region will converge at the terminal, and then travel up to the brain in one big wire. Since this system is not always perfect, the signal from one structure, such as a tooth, can be mixed up along the way, usually at the "junction box" where some of the wires come together before a larger wire is connected to the brain. By the time it gets to the brain, the information is understood as coming from another structure, the sinus for example, in the same region—what we would call "getting our wires crossed." The regions of the body that contain one set of mesh work of wires with one terminal are determined by where the cells of that region came from when you were just an embryo in the womb. Just like houses in a particular subdivision, the source of electricity for that subdivision would all come from the same substation.

Aside from the actual physical grouping of nerves, the processing of pain stimuli in our spinal cord and in our brain also likely play a part in the perception of referred pain. In this case, the pain felt may be some distance away from the actual injury site.

How is this important in our discussion of head and neck pain? Well, the majority of the pain nerves in the face, jaws and teeth all converge on one terminal. This terminal is called the trigeminal nucleus. The trigeminal nucleus is extremely important in the pain-transmission of the face, teeth, jaw and neck area. This area includes all the chewing muscles, some of the head-movement muscles, the TMJ, all the teeth, the sinuses and the bones of the upper and lower jaw.

What is also extremely interesting to note is that migraine headaches, which is generally accepted as a primary headache (a headache that has no other causes) also have pain that originate or passes through the trigeminal nerve. Therefore, the majority of head-pains, whether it is primary or secondary in nature, are the direct result of pain transmitted, altered, modified through the trigeminal nucleus.

Large part of a dentist's role is pain control, so our training in school and a large part of our clinical life are spent understanding and controlling sources of pain. The area of our interest is mostly inside the mouth, involving teeth and gums. According to one study in the USA, 16% of patients visit the dentist because of pain. Whenever we do a filling we need to "freeze" the tooth and gums in that area. So we know the anatomy and especially the nerves involved in this area. Coincidentally, the nerves that we "freeze" for pain control are part of the trigeminal nerve. Therefore, dental pain is often referred to other parts of the face and head, and vice versa, which are covered by the same trigeminal nerve.

There are many other examples of referred pain. The most common forms in this area of the body are exemplified by a condition called myofascial pain syndrome (MPS). MPS is a chronic pain disorder in which pressure on sensitive points in your muscles (trigger points) causes pain in seemingly unrelated parts of your body.

MPS typically occurs after a muscle or fascia has been over worked. This can be caused by repetitive motions used in jobs or hobbies or by stress-related muscle tension such as grinding or clenching of teeth. While nearly everyone has experienced muscle-tension pain, the discomfort associated with MPS persists or worsens.

The referred pain patterns in the head and neck region show that injuries in the muscles of chewing, and muscles used for head movements, mimic that of primary headaches and migraines. This is one of the major reasons why chronic headaches are not diagnosed and treated properly.

We want to know what can go wrong with the systems that cause pain (which were discussed in the previous chapter) and, more importantly, what can cause the kind of pain that will qualify as chronic headaches or migraines. The following is a chart of the types of orofacial pain (pain in the mouth, face and head). This is a very comprehensive chart put together by the International Association for the Study of Pain.

Table 1.

Neuralgias

- Acute herpes zoster
- Geniculate neuralgia (VII)
- Glossopharyngeal neuralgia (IX)
- Hypoglossal neuralgia (XII)
- Post-herpetic neuralgia
- Secondary neuralgias
- Short-lasting, unilateral, neuralgiform pain with conjunctival injection and tearing (SUNCT)
- Tolosa-Hunt syndrome
- Trigeminal neuralgia

Musculoskeletal pains

- Acute tension-type headache
- Chronic tension-type headache
- Crushing injury of head or face
- Rheumatoid arthritis of the temporomandibular joint
- Temporomandibular disorders (TMDs)

Primary Headaches

- Carotidynia
- Chronic paroxysmal hemicrania
- Classic migraine
- Cluster headache
- Common migraine
- Hemicrania continua
- Mixed headache
- Post-traumatic headache
- Temporal arteritis

Pains in the ear, nose and oral cavity

- Atypical odontalgia and facial pain
- Burning mouth syndrome
- Cracked tooth syndrome
- Diseases of the jaw
- Dry socket
- Frostbite of face
- Gingival disease
- Maxillary sinusitis
- Odontalgia
- Otitis media

Psychological pains

- Associated with depression
- Delusional or hallucinatory pain
- Hysterical, conversion or hypochondriacal pain

Examples of pain conditions that occur in the head and face. Some are extremely rare (e.g. Tolosa-Hunt syndrome) and are most likely to be seen only by neurologists or other pain specialists. Others are very common (acute tension-type headache, TMDs and odontalgias) in everyday dental practice. Note that the groupings are based on a mixture of e.g. regions, tissues and pain mechanisms. Modified from Merskey, H. and Bogduk, N. (Eds.) Classification of chronic pain. IASP Press: Seattle, 1994.

We will go over some of the more common conditions in this chart, and a couple that are not included on the chart. These would represent more than 90% of the head-pain experienced by chronic headache patients.

Temporomandibular Disorder (TMD)

The temporomandibular joint, what I've been referring to as TMJ, is the joint that hinges your jaw. You have two jaws—the upper jaw is called the maxilla, and the lower jaw is called the mandible. The upper jaw is fixed to the skull, while the lower jaw is the one that moves. The movement of the mandible is accomplished by a group of muscles (muscles of mastication), and the TMJ. This is a very unique and complex joint. The most unique features are:

1. It is the only bone in the body where the two joints (one on each side of the face) must work at the same time.
2. These joints rotate and slide forward out of the socket.
3. It is one of two joints in the body that has an articulating disk.

Temporomandibular Disorders (TMD) have a complex and poorly understood set of conditions. The main problems are pain in the jaw joint and surrounding tissues and limitation in jaw movement. Injuries and other conditions that routinely affect other joints in the body, such as arthritis, also affect the TMJ. One or both joints may be involved and, depending on the severity, can affect a person's ability to speak, chew, swallow, make facial expressions and even breathe. Also included under the heading of TMD are disorders involving the jaw muscles. These may accompany the jaw-joint problems or occur independently.

Approximately 12% of the population (or 35 million people) in the United States are affected by TMD at any given time. While both men and women experience these disorders, the majority of those seeking treatment are women in their childbearing years. Considering that 1 in 8 people have this problem at any given time, and an estimated up to 80% of the population will experience these symptoms at one point in their lives, this is an extremely common head-pain. The treatment for TMD is almost exclusively carried out by dentists.

Furthermore, scientists have found that most patients with TMD also experience painful conditions in other parts of the body. These conditions include chronic fatigue syndrome, chronic headache, fibromyalgia, irritable bowel syndrome, low back pain, sleep disorders, and others. Therefore, the diagnosis and treatment can become fairly complex, and a dentist must be involved.

Trigeminal neuralgia (TN)

Trigeminal neuralgia is considered one of the most painful afflictions known to man. The reason why we are talking about it is because it is one of the most common nerve conditions, and it affects the exact nerve that controls pain sensation in the oral and facial area, as discussed in the last chapter.

The typical or "classic" form of the disorder (called TN1) causes extreme, sporadic, sudden burning or shock-like facial pain in the areas of the face where the branches of the nerve are distributed—lips, eyes, nose, scalp, forehead, upper jaw and lower jaw. The pain episodes last from a few seconds to as long as two minutes. These attacks can occur in quick succession, on and off for as long as two hours. The atypical form of the disorder (called TN2), is characterized by constant aching, burning, stabbing pain of somewhat lower intensity than TN1. Both forms of pain may occur in the same person, sometimes at the same time.

The trigeminal nerve is one of 12 pairs of nerves that are attached to the brain. The nerve has three branches that conduct sensations from the upper, middle and lower portions of the face, as well as the oral cavity, to the brain (see Figure 1). More than one nerve branch can be affected by the disorder. On rare occasions, both sides of the face may be affected at different times in one individual, or even more rarely at the same time (called bilateral TN).

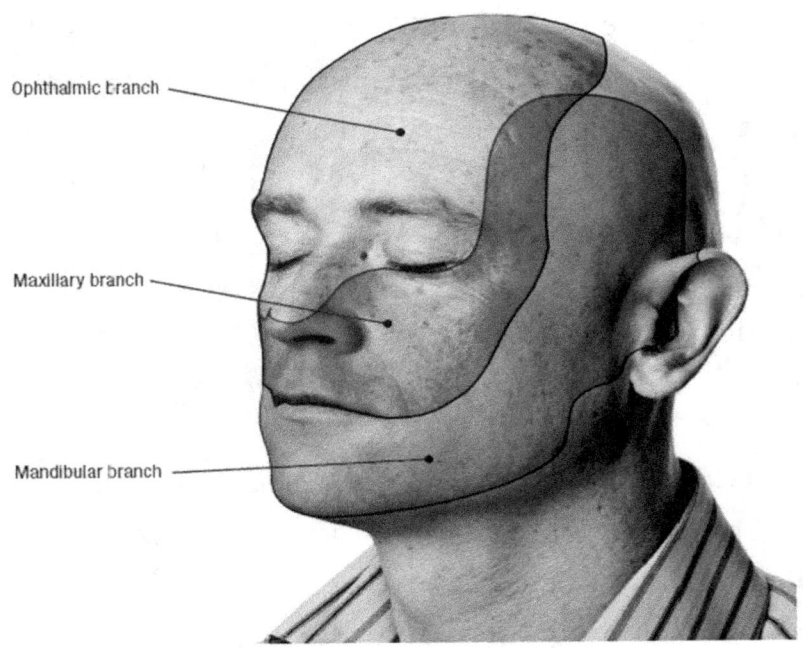

Ophthalmic branch

Maxillary branch

Mandibular branch

Figure 1. Distribution of the cranial nerve V: the ophthalmic nerve (V₁), the maxillary nerve (V₂), and the mandibular nerve (V₃).

[Figure 1: Distribution of the 5th Cranial Nerve: Disorders of the Maxillary and Mandibular Branches Can Present as a Toothache Causing Patients to Seek Dental Treatment.]

The intense flashes of pain can be triggered by vibration or contact with the cheek (such as when shaving, washing the face or applying makeup), brushing teeth, eating, drinking, talking or being exposed to the wind. People with TN avoid social contact and daily activities such as eating and talking because they fear an attack. Many have been known to lose their jobs because of the debilitating nature of the pain. Marriages have dissolved due to the difficulty of providing care and support to persons with TN. Pain from TN is frequently very isolating and depressing for the individual. Depression and sleep disturbance may render individuals more vulnerable to pain and suffering. Trigeminal neuralgia is often referred to as the "suicide disease" and many doctors consider it to be one of the most painful diseases known. Thus, there are individual, familial and societal costs of TN.

Because of overlapping symptoms and the large number of conditions that can cause facial pain, obtaining a correct diagnosis is difficult, but finding the cause of the pain is important as the treatments for different types of pain may differ. Trigeminal neuralgia occurs at a rate of less than 0.1% of the population, so it is considered a rare disease; however, it is one of the most common diseases of the nervous system.

Primary headaches

The definition of *headache* has been discussed in Chapter 3. Although we do not know all the origins of headaches, we do know that headaches often accompany other orofacial pain conditions.

Myofascial pain syndrome

Myofascial pain syndrome (MPS) is characterized by chronic pain in muscles and the layer of connective tissue covering and separating individual muscles, called *fascia*. The pain is due to knots in the muscles call *trigger points*, or constrictions in the fascia. Trigger points can be tender points in the muscles that produce pain in a particular muscle or cause pain at a location that is far away from the trigger point itself, which is a form of referred pain. Referred pain is discussed in the previous chapter. The common trigger points in particular muscles and their referred pain patterns are mapped out through the early works of Dr. Janet Travell in her groundbreaking work in 1942.

The causes of MPS are not fully documented or understood. This is not to deny the existence of the clinical phenomena themselves. Some systemic diseases, such as connective tissue disease, can cause MPS. Poor posture and emotional disturbance might also instigate or contribute to MPS. What it does mean is that MPS can contribute to head-pain conditions, further confusing the originating pain sources in such complex cases.

These are the common causes of pain in the head and face region. The pain these conditions cause often get confused with or mimics migraine headaches, or they will trigger or occur at the same time as migraine headaches. There are many other conditions on that list; however, they are relatively rare. The important thing to note is that half of the conditions on that list are primarily treated by a dentist, and 80% of the conditions by frequency of occurrence, fall under the scope of practice in dentistry.

Chapter 6

Secret #1: A Special Group of Sufferers—Dentomandibular Sensorimotor Dysfunction (DMSD)

"The expression of DMSD is chronic pain and stiffness of the head and neck area, transmitted through the trigeminal nerve as a result of imbalance of dental forces."

Ten signs or symptoms of DMSD:

1. Jaw clicking
2. Chronic headaches or migraines
3. Limited movement in the neck or jaw
4. Painful or sore muscles in the neck or jaw
5. Tooth fracture or excessive tooth wear
6. Grinding or clenching of teeth
7. Past history of trauma from car accident or sports injury
8. Repetitive strain injuries from work or hobbies
9. Poor sleep or sleep apnea

10. Ringing in your ear or vertigo

For many years now, dentists have been observing, studying and treating a number of these disorders causing orofacial pain. As mentioned in the last chapter, many of these conditions seem to have common causes rooted in information-processing of the trigeminal nerve and related cranial nerves. Now, the latest research in the neuroscience of the trigeminal nucleus bears out the observations, suspicions and treatment efforts of these dentists, so much so that we can now begin to group many of these disorders into a category that we call dentomandibular sensorimotor dysfunction (DMSD).

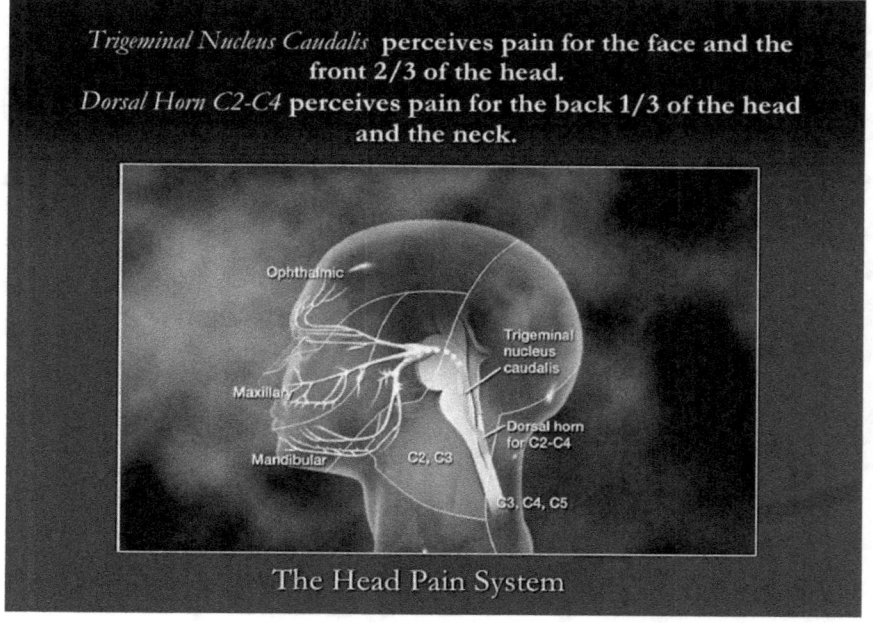

Trigeminal Nucleus Caudalis perceives pain for the face and the front 2/3 of the head.
Dorsal Horn C2-C4 perceives pain for the back 1/3 of the head and the neck.

The Head Pain System

DMSD is a medical condition that involves the muscles for chewing and neck movement, soft tissues, teeth, joints in the jaw and top three vertebrae of the neck (C1, C2, C3). There is a concentrated nerve center in this area called the trigeminal nucleus caudalis. This major pathway of nerves controls pain signals from the teeth, face, head and neck, and carries them to the brain. The expression of DMSD is chronic pain and stiffness of the head and neck area, transmitted through the trigeminal nerve as a result of imbalance of dental forces.

The dental foundation consists of teeth, muscles and joints in the dentofacial (head and neck) area. The dental foundation is considered to be out of balance when one or more of the following conditions apply:

- Advanced aging or disability of the muscles which open the jaw
- Movement or noises in the jaw joints which indicate the disks in the neck are moving, deformed or swollen
- Tooth wear or breakage
- Limited range of motion in the jaw and cervical (neck) spine
- Painful or sore head and/or neck muscles, with very sensitive spots (trigger points)

- Pain that stems from the trigeminocervical nucleus
- Any lifestyle limitation related to the teeth, muscles or joints of the head and neck

There are many symptoms associated with DMSD conditions. The most commonly reported are:

- Headache/migraine
- Chronic daily headache
- Tension-type headache
- Myofascial pain
- Tinnitus
- Temporomandibular joint disorder (TMJD)
- Toothaches
- Poor airway control
- Sleep/arousal disorder
- Changes in brain chemistry and neurotransmitter balance
- Bruxism
- Craze lines on teeth
- Tooth fracture/damage
- Unstable dental arch form
- Restricted range of motion and postural adaptations
- Clenching

- Abnormal tooth-wear patterns
- Malocclusion (a bite that is crooked, unbalanced and unstable)
- Non-productive jaw movements
- Degenerative joint disease

Traditional medicine does not cover all the areas that make up the dental foundation; therefore, individuals that experience chronic headaches or migraines without finding lasting relief, despite having been through assessments by medical doctors, may be suffering from DMSD. A recent development of objective tests and thorough gathering of past medical history can accurately identify this condition. What we found is that a large percentage of the chronic head-pain patients that have not been successfully treated by the conventional medical system would have major elements of DMSD condition. This observation bears out in the fact that when these patients come into our offices and are diagnosed with DMSD, up to 93% of them will respond positively to our treatment.

Dentists are widely regarded as doctors that fill cavities in teeth. However, the oral cavity is so much more complex than that, and the health of your teeth and gums directly affects the health of the rest of your body. It is good to recognize the importance of this fact, and of creating a whole different branch in our healthcare system devoted to its care. Unfortunately, the separation of medicine from dentistry created a large enough divide that knowledge and cooperation between the two professions at the clinical level became an obstacle in the treatment of a large majority of chronic head-pain patients. This is apparent in the fact that these patients with problems in both the medical and dental fields are rarely treated by the same practitioner, and parts of necessary diagnosis and treatment can be missed. This is the heart of the problem we are dealing with in this book.

1. There is a large group of patients with head-pain being treated by either medical doctors or dentists where traditional treatment in either field alone cannot offer the entire solution.
2. These patients have multiple factors that fall into the field of medicine and dentistry, making their condition very complex.
3. This is why there is an epidemic proportion of the population with chronic head-pain.
4. Groups of pain conditions in the head and neck areas are controlled by the trigeminal nucleus; in fact this would include 80% of the orofacial pain conditions by frequency of occurrence.

5. By grouping them together we have created a new identity called dentomandibular sensorimotor dysfunction, or DMSD.

6. We need to combine diagnosis and treatment modalities from both advanced dentistry and rehabilitative medicine to treat these conditions.

7. 93% success rate in reducing the frequency, intensity and duration of pain when properly diagnosed.

8. Most of the chronic head-pain patients that have been through years of medical and alternative medicine treatments without success would likely fall within this category.

Chapter 7

Secret #2: A Bucket Full of Reasons

"The things that fill up in the bucket are factors that contribute to chronic- pain situations. As the factors are filling up the bucket, your tolerance to pain becomes less, until the bucket is full, and pain becomes constant."

One sunny Saturday morning, I was busy at work when Rick walked in for his scheduled new patient consultation. My assistant seated him in my consultation room and asked him to fill out the extensive medical history and questionnaire that we provide to all the new head-pain patients. When I walked into the room, I saw a stoic young man in his 20s, dressed in a football jersey and baggy shorts, obviously an ex-athlete, may have starred on his high school football team. Those days had since passed him by, and he was now about 50 pounds over fighting weight, and not particularly comfortable in his new skin.

I began my consultation in my usual manner, by greeting him and starting the process like an interview. Getting the story behind the journey that led him to my office was paramount in the initial diagnosis. I started off slow to get a feel for his mindset. I began by asking him the usual simple questions of who referred him to us and what his symptoms were, etc. He answered my questions with short, abrupt answers, in a somewhat disinterested tone. Most of the time, patients are more than interested in telling their story, because this is the agony of what they have been living with for the past number of months or years. The hours of their days are filled with thoughts of how to minimize their pain. What do they have to do to get through the day. What medication to take at which time, what activities will bring about or exacerbate their pain. When they have any exciting plans or events coming up, they are always afraid of another round of pain that will put them in a dark room and cause them to miss some of life's more important moments. They are more than preoccupied—they are slaves to the pain. So usually they want to talk about it, afraid that any detail they leave out may be of crucial importance to solving their problem.

Rick was different; right from the start he seemed disinterested, and he answered questions reluctantly, almost guarded. Once I read the situation, I quickly stopped the interview.

Rick and others like him fall into a different, less common group of patients. He viewed me with skepticism and distrust. He was torn between desperately wanting to finally find the solution to his pain and protecting himself from yet another round of disappointments. In his mind, he could not let himself hang his hope on another quack that claimed to be able to help him, only to have his hopes crushed and the pain continue to take its toll on his health and his mind. He was too young to lose hope.

I read through the questionnaire he had filled out. He was a 29-year-old male working in the venture capital business. An ex-football player and a regular gym rat, he enjoyed action sports and was not afraid to take risks. Contact sports, body building and gambling on small business start-ups fulfilled his passions. That was until the day that he was hurt in a car crash. Now he was in constant pain, couldn't work out, gained 50 pounds of fat. He was afraid that he wouldn't be able to reach his goals in life and enjoy the fruits of his labor.

I saw on the forms that the car accident happened over a year ago, and that he had found us searching on the Web. I knew that my clinic was relatively new in the city; it was not part of the normal medical referral destinations.

Since he was reluctant to tell me his story, I decided to tell it to him myself.

I said, "You were hurt in a car accident. At the time of the accident, you were quickly taken to a hospital. They did a detailed examination of your physical condition, including a thorough examination, took X-rays, CT scan, even an MRI if it was necessary. Any cuts or broken bones were efficiently taken care of, including any necessary surgery. They prescribed pain meds, anti-inflammatories, and any other medications that you needed at the time. They sent you home at this point and told you to follow up with your family doctor. You were sore, but counted yourself lucky, because all the injuries seemed to be recovering. You went to your family doctor, if you had one, and they told you to rest and you would be fine.

As days turned into weeks, the initial rapid recovery slowed down. Some of the aches and pains went away, but other problems started to appear. Your back and neck started to hurt in places that hadn't hurt before. You started to get headaches, maybe jaw pains. You went back to your family doctor, who prescribed you more meds and set you up to see a physiotherapist, telling you this was the normal recovery process. The physiotherapy took longer to see results—in the meantime, your headaches got worse, and you fatigued easily, wanted to stay in bed or curl up in dark places. You couldn't work properly. You went back to your doctor again, with the new symptoms, and again your doctor upped or changed your medication, and perhaps sent you to go see a medical specialist. You saw an ENT doctor or a neurologist or both. They did not find anything definitive. More tests were done, and they ruled out brain damage or infections.

So you stayed on the meds, and quit seeing the physiotherapist. You started to have dark thoughts, became more antisocial, preferring to stay home and wait out the pain. The side effects of the meds got you back to the doctor; you complained that they were not working and the side effects were worse than the pain at times. New drugs were tried, maybe even antidepressants. Weeks turned into months, and you decided that all those meds were making you worse, so you quit them all—or maybe you just wanted to take more of certain ones. Maybe you became addicted to some.

If you were a fighter—and I think you are—you took matters into your own hands. You started to seek out alternative treatments. Your family and friends made suggestions; you may have tried massage, chiropractor, Rolfing, IMS, acupuncture, craniosacral therapy or any of the combinations. They did not work, or worked only partially and did not last. Finally, you found me on the Net late one night surfing because you couldn't sleep. You did not really believe in what you saw on my Webpage, but the patient testimonies got you interested. You didn't believe that a dentist could solve problems that your doctor and all those medical specialists couldn't. However, you owed it to yourself to find the solution, because you're not a quitter and not ready to give up just yet.

"That's how you came to be here today."

Rick's eyes grew round and lit up, and as I went through the details of his tortuous journey into despair, his jaw dropped. How could I have gotten all that from his few yes and no answers? At this point, he became friendlier and more cooperative. I was able to complete my initial physical examinations and assessment. He told me that he has a lawyer that we needed to get involved. We shook hands at the end of the examination, and he walked out with a little more hope.

What I told that young man, or a version of it, is something I have seen all too frequently. Complex chronic pain patients go through this journey seeking for help in all the unlikely places. They usually do this alone, or if they are lucky, they have a support system of loyal friends and family. But it is like searching for the answer in the dark, randomly and desperately trying anything they come across.

Our medical system is great at assessing and treating acute, obvious injuries. Emergency rooms are full of people, and the demand on this system makes them work fast and efficiently. They will get you in and get you out quickly. After you are out, however, is when the ball is dropped. Our bodies have the innate ability to repair themselves. When the initial damage is repaired, most of the time we will recover. But some of the time, hidden injuries or previous imbalances in our bodies prevent a full recovery. Conditions like whiplash syndrome can take weeks or even months to fully manifest. Trauma in one area of the body overloads another area, which causes symptoms to appear elsewhere. Family physicians—where comprehensive care is founded—are becoming a rare species. Most people go to walk-in clinics for their sporadic medical care, where complex chronic pain, with its multiple elusive causes, takes too much time in cough-and-cold practices. Treating symptoms with drugs is becoming the solution, instead of time-consuming detective work required to rout out all the causes.

The root of these cases is usually multifaceted. Some factors relate directly to the initial cause, others are cascading events and some are even more elusive. Chronic pain is rarely due to a single cause, because if that were the case, someone would have figured it out already and you would be cured. I explain this process to my patients with my Bucket analogy.

Bucket Analogy

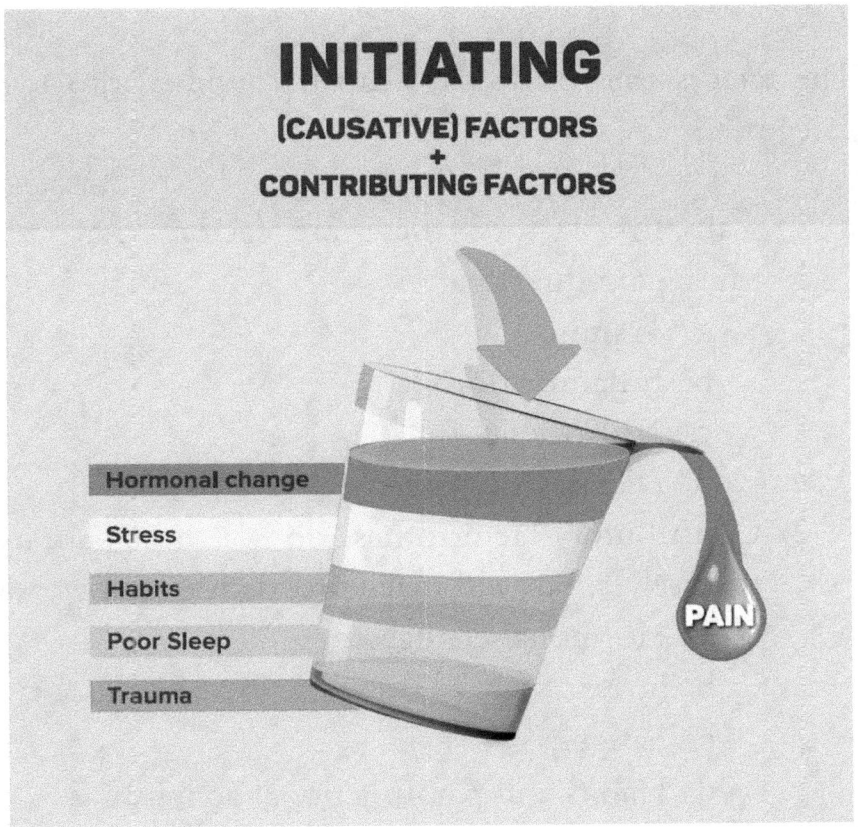

The bucket represents your body's ability to control pain. The things that fill up in the bucket are factors that contribute to chronic-pain situations. As the factors are filling up the bucket, your tolerance to pain becomes less, until the bucket is full and pain becomes constant. You may remove one or more of these factors and feel a little better; but it would be very easy for the bucket to spill over again and for you to return to the pain state.

The factors that cause pain can be divided into two categories:

1) Causative factors: these are factors that can cause pain directly
    a. Trauma
    b. Inflammation
    c. Neurogenic
    d. Diseases/disorders
2) Contributory factors: these do not cause pain by themselves, but will make preexisting pain worse
    a. Hormonal changes
    b. Stress
    c. Fatigue
    d. Habits and parafunctional activity
    e. Medication side effects
    f. Psychological changes/disorder
    g. Congenital defects

Therefore, the more factors you can identify and solve, the less you will have in the "bucket," the better your chances are of keeping the pain away.

A good example of this multifactorial pain complex that you may be familiar with is whiplash syndrome.

The exact injury mechanism that causes whiplash injuries is unknown. A whiplash injury from an automobile accident is called a cervical acceleration-deceleration injury. This is a situation where the spine, with the head at the top of it, is whipped through a quick acceleration at impact. The head, which is at the end of the whip, will snap like a whip under these quick changes in speed. The strain on the ligaments in the neck and other tendons and soft tissues in the head and neck causes injury.

Whiplash may be caused by any motion similar to a rear-end collision in a motor vehicle, such as on a rollercoaster or other rides at an amusement park, sports injuries such as football or soccer accidents, other modes of transportation such as airplane travel, or from being hit, kicked or shaken.

Whiplash-associated disorders sometimes include injury to the base of the brain. In a severe cervical acceleration–deceleration syndrome, a brain injury known as a coup-contrecoup injury occurs. A coup-contrecoup injury occurs when the brain is accelerated into the cranium as the head and neck hyperextend, and is then accelerated into the other side as the head and neck rebound to hyper-flexion or neutral position. This is also the same injury mechanism as a concussion.

Whiplash is one of the most common nonfatal car crash injuries. More than one million whiplash injuries occur each year due to car crashes. This is an estimate, because not all cases of whiplash are reported. "Freeman and co-investigators estimated that 6.2% of the US population have late whiplash syndrome." The majority of cases occur in patients in their late forties.

As you can see, pain-process in whiplash syndrome is usually not from just injury to one area. Neck muscle strain, ligament sprain, TMD, psychological factors— all play a role. The progression of this disorder can include some or all of these components, and the speed at which the syndrome evolves can vary from days to week to months. The areas covered can include neck muscles, jaw muscles, cervical vertebrae, the TMJ, teeth, nervous system. In order to treat this effectively, you must first find all the problems and treat each one individually and collectively.

The most obvious symptom of whiplash syndrome is pain; however, it is difficult to determine the specific cause of the pain, since causative factors in this case may be direct injury to the ligaments, tendons, muscles, joints, brain injury, concussion, etc. Perpetuating factors can include poor bite balance, preexisting TMD, psychological factors, myofascial pain syndrome, hormonal changes and many others. In order to properly treat these patients, you need to determine what is in the "bucket" and then reduce them as much as possible.

You may notice that, as in the whiplash syndrome, there is no one cause for your syndrome; in fact, the symptoms and causes are many and ill-defined—they overlap and include many other dysfunctions. Dentomandibular sensorimotor dysfunction acts the same way. It includes many of the same symptoms as the whiplash syndrome, myofascial pain syndrome, temporomandibular dysfunction and chronic headaches. It is safe to say that many of the factors causing pain conditions overlap and can occur at the same time. In addition, each patient has their own unique set of perpetuating factors and habits. The single most common initiating cause for DMSD patients' pain becoming chronic and complex is motor vehicle accidents, followed by work-related injuries. Preexisting conditions from lists of common orofacial pain conditions may also exist to varying degrees, creating each patient's unique and complicated pain profile.

Treatment by experts in the medical field rarely consider areas in and around the oral cavity. Therefore, many of the imbalances described in DMSD are not addressed, and their "buckets" are still full.

Chapter 8

Secret #3: Discovering the Problems

"The reason why some practitioners have failed in these cases is because not enough of the pain factors have been diagnosed and dealt with. The imbalance of the dental foundation, muscles, joints and oral cavity, is still present; therefore, many of the treatments can only provide temporary relief."

"There are many problems that only a dentist can diagnose such as toothaches, gum disease, oral habits, and poor bite that can cause pain in the facial area. There are other problems in the oral cavity that require other medical or dental specialists to treat but can be diagnosed by a dentist, such as airway problems, sleep apnea, enlarged or infected tonsils and adenoids, nasal obstruction, allergies problems, sinus infections ..."

1) History
2) Must have medical backup
3) Inside and out
4) Muscle palpation
5) TMJ assessment

6) Dental assessment

7) Dental force analysis

8) Range of motion

As previous chapters have suggested, dentists are often the best choice for assessment and treatment of head-pain. Not only are we well versed in the anatomy and physiology of this area, we alone among the entire healthcare profession are able to combine expertise in medicine, physical therapy, rehabilitative therapy and advance dentistry for treatments in the head and neck areas. This is not to say that we should be the only healthcare providers to treat all headaches—far from it! There are causes to headaches that only a medical professional can diagnose and treat. However, they are a relatively small percentage by occurrence.

The typical patient that I have seen in my practice suffers from chronic pain. As described in the story about Rick, they have the following profile:

1. Pain condition anywhere from 3 months to 25 years or more

2. Have seen family physician plus other specialists

3. Have not had lasting success with any conventional treatment

4. Have tried alternative healthcare
5. Have tried many different drugs; either the drugs have not worked and have too many side effects to continue using, or they are on so many different drugs that they are afraid to get off of them
6. Symptoms involve many areas of the head and neck that elude simple diagnosis

To properly diagnose these patients, we must start with the pain history. This part takes anywhere from a half hour to an hour, and is extremely important in the diagnosis of their condition. The reason why some practitioners have failed in these cases is because not enough of the pain factors have been diagnosed and dealt with. The imbalance of the dental foundation, muscles, joints and oral cavity is still present; therefore, many of the treatments can only provide temporary relief.

To thoroughly diagnose any less common but critical dysfunctions and diseases, the patient may need to be referred to our medical colleagues for assessment when indicated. As I had mentioned before, most of the chronic head-pain patients have already consulted their family physician or other medical specialists, which should be revealed in their health history.

Following the patient history interview, we continue with the clinical evaluation.

Physical exam

A thorough clinical exam of the head and neck is needed. This would include palpating the muscles of the head and neck as well as those used for chewing, looking for knots and trigger points, checking the TMJ for joint sounds and pain and restrictions.

Oral exam

As mentioned before, many problems inside the oral cavity can cause pain, due to the fact that the nerves that transmit pain inside the mouth are the same pain nerves for the rest of the face and neck. There are many problems that only a dentist can diagnose such as toothaches, gum disease, oral habits and poor bite that can cause pain in the facial area. There are other problems in the oral cavity that require other medical or dental specialists to treat but can be diagnosed by a dentist, such as airway problems, sleep apnea, enlarged or infected tonsils and adenoids, nasal obstruction, allergies problems, sinus infections, among others.

Radiographic exam

Dentists regularly use X-rays and CT scans for diagnosing problems in the head and mouth region.

Radiographs can reveal diseases in teeth, jaws and joints. Orthodontists use these on a routine basis to look at the balance of bone and teeth structures. These techniques are also used in assessing overall balance and health of the dental foundation.

Dental force scans

Excessive force due to poor bite, injured muscles or unbalanced joints is critical in pain conditions. A dental force analysis is the best method in determining these force outliers. A functional recording of bite in action, such as chewing or biting, allows us to diagnose force imbalance that static exams do not. While this is a relatively new and less common diagnostic tool even in dentistry, nevertheless it is the gold standard in dental force analysis. The use of this technology in headache diagnosis is critical, since all excessive force in this area causes overloading of the system, leading to injury of one of the structures and ultimately pain.

Range-of-motion assessment

The cervical range-of-motion test is a standardized test with quantifiable results that give us an idea of the disability. Any restriction in the neck's movements can indicate injury to specific muscles and joints. Although it does not indicate pain, the identification of the area of restriction, together with a physical examination of the individual muscles and soft tissue, will give us a good picture of the injury pattern. This will lead to treatment directed to their rehabilitation.

In Chapter 5 we examined an extensive list of all the forms of head and neck pains. On that list, there are some diseases and disorders—such as ones originating in the nervous system, or caused by tumors or vascular diseases—that belong purely in the realm of specialized medicine. After all, we would not want to mistaken a headache caused by a brain tumor for one that is caused by tense muscles. However, looking at the list of pain-causing problems, we find that 80% or more of the individual problems are right in the wheelhouse of a properly trained dentist. I have emphasized that there is extra training required for dentists to become familiar and able to detect and treat this type of chronic head-pain patient.

The design of our assessment protocol is to tease out all the areas of possible pain production. This thorough examination covers all the areas of head and neck and oral cavity. The results give us a list of probable causes of the head-pain. As previously mentioned, the Bucket analogy dictates that we need to find as many of the factors as possible to reduce or eliminate pain on a long-term basis. At the end of this examination, we are able to create a list of problems that covers diseases and disorders spanning the field of medicine and dentistry which can cause pain. With this list, a plan can be created that will address as many of the problems in the "bucket" as possible, in order to achieve effective and lasting results.

Chapter 9

Secret #4: Finding a Solution That Lasts

"It is the art and science of properly identifying the source and location of injury together with removing the obstacles and boosting our healing powers that make us a 'healers.' It is our compassion and perseverance in gaining more knowledge and expanding our treatment methods that make us a great 'healers.' "

"... combination of advanced dentistry techniques and sports rehabilitation—derived therapies used in treating dental force imbalances ... This rehabilitative method resulted in dentists reporting 93% success rate in providing patients with real, lasting relief from their pain symptoms."

1) Muscle and soft tissue rehabilitation
   a. In-office therapy
      i. Ultrasound
      ii. Manual manipulation
      iii. Micro-current
      iv. Cold laser therapy
2) TMD treatment

  a. Oral appliances

  b. Short-term medication

  c. Exercises

3) Bite imbalances

  a. Dental disease control

  b. Bite force balancing

  c. Braces

  d. New fillings or teeth replacements

4) In-home care program

  a. Stretching and exercises

  b. Natural anti-inflammatories

  c. Psychological/stress management

  d. Sleep management

When I made the connection between chronic headaches and all the oral facial pain I had treated as a dental specialist that day in front of the booth at a dental conference, a whole new world opened up to me. I saw that there is no clear line that delineates the pain that we treat as dentists and the pain medical doctors treat on a daily basis. I began to take courses and learn different techniques that different healthcare professionals provide. I learned about what physical therapists do for injuries to muscles and joints in other parts of the body. I observed and learned the techniques of massage therapists. I spoke to my colleagues in chiropractic science. I even started to examine alternative medicine such as naturopathic medicine and traditional Chinese medicine.

During the summer of the third year of my dental training, I participated in a World Health Organization program that provided scholarly exchange of information between Canada and China. Participants were arranged to spend two weeks to a year in an academic institution of our choice to study our field of interest. I was already in the healthcare field, so I decided to learn more about the ancient art of acupuncture. I knew at the time that acupuncture was used to cure many ailments through the use of needles. The acupuncture needles along different meridians on the body could control, regulate and heal injuries and diseases in other parts of the body. The other important use of acupuncture that interested me was in the area of pain control, and this was where I concentrated my studies. I spent three months' time in which I spent six days a week in the classroom in the mornings and in the hospital treating patients in the afternoons. The experience gave me a greater appreciation for the complexity of our body, and the mysterious ways we can stimulate and regulate our body's ability to heal. This appreciation for the alternative serves me well now as I look to expand my scope of understanding in complex pain control.

In the field of Western medicine, I learned from the area of rehabilitative medicine. Since a large percentage of the complex chronic pain patients have their problems originate from traumatic events, the imbalances in their system are usually from undiagnosed and untreated injuries. I asked myself, "Who on Earth receives the best rehabilitative care?" My answer? Professional athletes. They are paid millions of dollars to perform; therefore, it stands to reason that they get the most technologically advanced treatment for recovery. Have you heard of a football player who has broken a leg or torn a shoulder being able to recover and come back within weeks of the injury to perform at the height of their abilities again? Well, I can tell you that when I damaged my knee, it took me two months to see a knee specialist, and another three months to get an MRI done—and that's before the rehab even began. The technology is there, we just have to get access to it and learn how to apply it to our specific needs. We now employ ultrasound, micro-current, TENs, intramuscular stimulation, acupressure, manual manipulation, cold laser, and many other technologies and techniques which have been available to athletes of the highest level, and applied them to the treatment of chronic head-pain.

The treatment of chronic pain in the head and neck region is made more difficult by the close proximity of structures of our senses. The nose, ears, mouth and eyes are very close together, and the different disorders causing pain that occur in each structure can easily overlap with one another. The expertise for pain control in the oral cavity and TMJ area belongs to the dental field. We are able to selectively bring the most effective treatment modality from dentistry to the equation. The goal is the same—we use dental appliances and techniques first to control and eliminate pain, and then further rehabilitation to eliminate any imbalances and restore health.

One of the first things you learn as a "healer" is that doctors do not actually "heal" patients. We are not magicians, whereby we can wave a magic wand and make injuries or diseases disappear! We are merely "facilitators"; your body is gifted with the ability to heal itself, but sometimes the cause of injury is not removed or damage is too extensive for the body to have a chance to heal. Our jobs as doctors are to identify the causes of injury, remove them and allow the body to heal itself. Sometimes the body is too weak or deficient in some way to complete the healing, so we must utilize techniques or technology to boost its natural abilities. We must work on both sides of the equation to maximize our chances at successfully treating difficult cases.

As I was studying the ancient art of acupuncture, I asked myself how sticking a bunch of needles in our bodies can cure so many ailments. The answer was found in the fact that the needles stimulate our body's natural healing powers. By trial and error, over thousands of years, we discovered the secret of deftly positioned needles triggering a cascade of physiological changes which increase production of chemicals or cells, thereby leading to your body healing itself. The principles of healing remain the same; the use of technology, in the right situations, has allowed us to boost our ability to heal even more.

A cautionary word about medication use in these patients and in general: some medications that deal specifically with an identifiable condition, such as the use of anticonvulsants in trigeminal neuralgia patients, are advisable. However, most painkillers such as opioids, anti-inflammatories, muscle relaxants, sedatives, etc. should be used on a very short-term basis. They are great in the initial phase of treatment to reduce pain and relax the patient so normal healing response of the body can occur. When the body cannot overcome the injury process, long-term use of these medications will not help healing, and will only mask the symptoms at best. In fact, long-term use of some medication can hurt the body with side effects, and some drugs such as opioids have serious addictive properties. Another common complication of long-term drug use is the rebound effect. In terms of pain, the medication overuse can actually become pain-producing and the primary reason for its propagation.

It is the art and science of properly identifying the source and location of injury together with removing the obstacles and boosting our healing powers that make us "healers." It is our compassion and perseverance in gaining more knowledge and expanding our treatment methods that make us great "healers."

Once the type of headache pain and extent of dental foundation imbalance is determined, treatment options are discussed. Historically, the treatments for headache pain included one or a combination of herbal remedies, stress-reduction exercises, massage, acupuncture, non-steroidal anti-inflammatory drugs (NSAID), narcotic pain relievers, anti-seizure medications, chiropractic adjustments, antidepressants or sedatives. Now, by using the combination of advanced dentistry techniques and sports rehabilitation–derived therapies used in treating dental force imbalances in dental headache care, we can reduce or eliminate the long-term use of medications and their side effects. This rehabilitative method resulted in dentists reporting 93% success rate in providing patients with real, lasting relief from their pain symptoms. The methods used control muscle force and force balance, restore proper function and range of motion and change the way the brain perceives stimuli so pain levels, dysfunction and improper muscle activity return to normal. By balancing the muscles, joints and teeth, and controlling the way the body feels pain in the head and neck areas, long-lasting pain relief can finally be achieved.

Chapter 10

Secret #5: Dentists, the Natural Choice

"... since many of the pain conditions in this area refer pain from one area to another, making them more complex, dentists have the responsibility to diagnose and treat these chronic pain conditions. Therefore, dentists must be one of the first choices for patients who are seeking solutions to their chronic pain conditions."

1) Dentists are the only healthcare practitioners that can work inside and outside of the oral cavity.

2) Like medical doctors, dentists have extensive fundamental medical training in the anatomy and physiology of the head and neck areas.

3) Dentists can prescribe drugs, use physical therapy, massage, intramuscular stimulation, sport-rehabilitation techniques, acupuncture, devices inside the mouth, all within one office by one practitioner.

4) The diagnosis and treatment of 80% of the pain found in the head and neck region falls within the scope of dental practices.

The American Dental Association's definition of what is "under the care of dentists" states that our expertise lies not only in treating the teeth and gums, but also in caring for the muscles of the head, neck and jaw, as well as, the nervous system of these areas.

According to the International Association for the Study of Pain, "In addition to the diagnosis and treatment of acute dental pain and pathology, such as that which may arise from trauma, infection, or other odontogenic origin, the orofacial pain dentist has the responsibility to diagnose and treat nonodontogenic orofacial pain—pain that is often chronic and persistent, multifactorial and complex, distressing, and debilitating."

The study goes on, "The complexity of the spectrum of orofacial pain disorders is compounded by the close proximity of numerous anatomical structures, including the eyes, nose, teeth, tongue, sinuses, ears, regional muscles, and the temporomandibular joints. These structures may be the source of facial pain that can refer to nearby but uninvolved areas. For example, it is not uncommon for cross-referral to occur between headaches and other orofacial pain conditions."

What this means is that because dentists are the primary healthcare practitioners capable of diagnosing problems both inside the mouth and the structures around the face and head, and since many of the pain conditions in this area refer pain from one area to another, making them more complex, dentists have the responsibility to diagnose and treat these chronic pain conditions. Therefore, dentists must be one of the first choices for patients who are seeking solutions to their chronic pain conditions.

From my experience, dentists are generally diagnosticians, artists and technicians all wrapped up in one. They are used to taking the patients from the initial consultation to the end treatment results all in their own clinic. This is a little different than in the medical system where the family physicians are the gatekeepers to the various avenues of treatment for specific conditions and diseases. Each condition or disease is diagnosed by a different specialist, and often times the treatment is then performed by another practitioner, such as physiotherapist, massage therapist or other technologist. Continuity may be lost in this process and gaps in treatment can be the end result.

Most dentists are technology-savvy. We are used to having an assortment of high-tech equipment in our office. We tend to use technology in our treatment process, and are generally interested in keeping up with its use. The success in the treatment outlined in the previous chapter demands the use of the latest dental and sports/rehab–medicine technology. I have personally invested considerable resources in acquiring these technologies and eagerly learned the proper use of them because of my familiarity with equipment and technology used in dentistry. My knowledge of the rehabilitation of muscles and joints of the head and neck is a natural extension of my knowledge used in dentistry.

Remember Dennis? He was one of my patients that kick started my search into head-pain control and treatment. His situation was desperate, with no real focus or goals toward rehabilitation. As we learned more and more about diagnostic techniques and treatment regimen, Dennis became one of our first test-cases. Over a course of nine weeks, using the techniques discussed in previous chapters, we systematically reduced or eliminated injuries to his neck muscles, rehabilitated his TMJ and slowly weaned him off of any medication dependency. We also taught him how to control his pain and recognize what his symptoms mean, and gave him a home-care regimen that gave him control over the injury and pain he was experiencing. His pain went away, and we are now rebalancing his bite so that he can enjoy long-lasting pain-free days.

It is extremely satisfying to be able to journey through such a life-changing experience with your patients; to see the transformation over many months from a person in the depths of despair to be reborn in rigors of life and hope. In particular, I truly enjoyed the aspect of hands-on multifaceted treatment procedures performed each week, sometimes taking two steps forward and one step back, but always with a goal and improvement in sight, and being able to be intimately involved in the journey to health.

Dennis is still coming to see me on a regular basis, and he relayed to me that he has pain about two times a month, which he is able to manage on his own. He also has been able to get and keep a job for the last six months. The change in him is clearly visible—there is life back in his demeanor and the future once again is something to which he can look forward to.

Chapter 11

Conclusion.

1. Eighty percent of head-pain is caused by injury.
2. Injury can be from diseases or trauma.
3. Most macrotrauma is caused by car accidents, sports or work-related accidents.
4. Microtrauma is due to habits, posture and work.
5. Other pain conditions causing or exacerbating head-pain include injury to teeth, gum, bite, sinus, TMJ and other orofacial structures.
6. Injury in the head and neck areas causes instability and imbalance.
7. The injuries and imbalances cause pain that is transmitted, altered, or modified by the trigeminal nucleus.
8. Dentists are the best healthcare provider to assess and treat this type of injury in the head and neck areas.
9. Treatment will include rehabilitative therapy inside and outside the mouth.
10. When properly assessed, our treatment success-rate is greater than 93% in reducing the intensity, frequency and duration of chronic pain.

Now that you have a deeper understanding of the sources of headaches and migraines, you can see how dentists are the obvious choice for diagnosing and treating your head-pain. I do have to emphasize that extra training would be needed by dentists to bolster our fundamental understanding in the realm of pain control and rehabilitative science in order to effectively serve patients in this complex field.

One emerging area that is coming to focus for the medical field is the area of obstructive sleep apnea (OSA). If you have not heard of it, you will definitely hear about it soon. OSA is a condition in which a person stops breathing during sleep. The stoppage in breathing can be a few seconds to as long as over a minute. This can happen multiple times in an hour, and hundreds of times in a night. Since your body does not receive adequate oxygen, it cannot function properly. The stoppage in breathing also wakes you up from your sleep. When this is happening hundreds of times a night, you do not get any real deep sleep at all—ever! The toll on your health is tremendous, and it is a life-threatening condition on so many levels; anything from heart disease to falling asleep at the wheel while driving. It is estimated that over 20% of

Americans over 50 years old are afflicted with this condition.

We know even less about how it affects children. Sleep apnea in infants was first identified in 1975 as sudden infant death syndrome and OSA. Today, OSA in children is recognized as the most severe form of the disease continuum of Sleep Disordered Breathing. Much research is being done, and the results point to multiple conditions, including snoring, labored breathing during sleep, high blood pressure and bedwetting. Children with OSA can often be underweight and may not have daytime sleepiness. Instead, they could have attention-deficient/hyperactivity disorder (ADHD). Left untreated, OSA has been shown to affect school performance and intellectual function, especially short-term memory and concentration ability. Interestingly, the vast majority of kids diagnosed with ADHD—when treated for sleep apnea, their ADHD symptoms disappear completely!

Since sleep apnea is an airway disorder that involves the tongue falling back into your throat, one of the most effective methods of control is through an appliance in your mouth. This is completely in the realm of dental professionals. Fortunately, dentists have become very involved in the research and treatment of this condition, and have made considerable progress in identifying and treating these patients. Interestingly, one of the most common features of these patients is daytime headaches and migraines.

Our professional mandate specifies that we have the proper training for diagnosing and treating conditions not just inside the oral cavity but muscles, joints and soft tissues of the head, neck and jaw, and the nervous system associated with these tissues. More and more dentists are becoming serious about treating these life-altering conditions; you owe it to yourself to seek out a qualified dentist for your head-pain today and get your life back.

Bibliography

1. Fernández-de-las-Peñas, Cuadrado, Arendt-Nielsen, Simons, Pareja. "Myofascial Trigger Points and Sensitization: An Updated Pain Model for Tension-Type Headache." Cephalalgia. May 2007: 383–393.
2. Miles, Nauntofte, Svensson, ed. Clinical Oral Physiology. Quintessence Publishing Co., 2004.
3. Temporomandibular Disorder. International Association for the Study of Pain, 2013.
4. Orofacial Pain. International Association for the Study of Pain, 2013.
5. Neurovascular Orofacial Pain. International Association for the Study of Pain, 2013.
6. Horst, Cunha-Cruz, Zhou, Manning, DeRouen. "Prevalence of pain in the orofacial regions in patients visiting general dentists in the Northwest Practice-based REsearch Collaborative in Evidence-based DENtistry research network." J of the Am Dental Assoc. October 2015: 721–728.
7. Murinova, Krashin. "Chronic Daily Headache." Phys Med Rehabil Clin N Am. 2015: 375–389.
8. DiMatteo, Montgomery, ed. Understanding, Assessing and Treating Dentomandibular

Sensorimotor Dysfunction. Dental Resource, Inc. 2012.

9. Fernandez. "Referred pain areas of active myofascial trigger points in head and neck and shoulder muscles in chronic tension-type headaches." J Body Mov Ther. Oct 2010: 391–396.

If you enjoyed this book and would like to be on the list for the prerelease of our next book,

Obstructive Sleep Apnea: Hidden Secrets of a Killer Disease,

please email us at dr.wangpacificwest@gmail.com.

In the meantime, turn the page for an exclusive first look!

This next book is co-authored with Dr. Kevin Lee, DDS MSc.

Obstructive Sleep Apnea: Secrets of a Hidden Killer Disease

Obstructive Sleep Apnea

Obstructive sleep apnea (OSA) is a medical syndrome that causes the breathing to become very shallow or completely stopped during sleep. OSA happens when something partially or completely blocks the airway during sleep. This could be due to malfunctioning of the airway muscles to keep the airway open, and/or abnormality in the structures surrounding the airway, making the airway smaller than usual. When OSA happens, the lung does not receive enough air, resulting in lack of oxygen to the rest of the body and the brain. Eventually, the brain wakes the body up from the sleep to activate the diaphragm and the chest muscles, and breathing usually resumes with a loud gasp, snort, or body jerk. The body and brain then falls back to sleep, and the whole process repeats itself. Patients with OSA may not realize that their sleep had been interrupted, but they typically will wake up 5-15 times an hour. Patients with severe form of the disease will wake up almost every minute!

How common is it?

Obstructive sleep apnea is common. In a review article published by American College of Physicians, it was reported that for white adults with an average body weight (BMI between 25 to 28 kg/m^2), 1 in 5 has mild OSA (an apnea–hypopnea index of 5 or greater); and 1 in 15 has moderate disease (an apnea-hypopnea index of 15 or greater). However, 75-80% of OSA patients were undiagnosed. Among those who were diagnosed, less than 25% of those diagnosed have been successfully treated.

Who is at risk for OSA?

Being Male. Men are 2-3 times more likely to have OSA than women. Postmenopausal women have increased risk for moderate OSA, an effect that hormone replacement therapy may reverse.

Being Obese. Approximately 70% of OSA patients are obese with body mass index (BMI) greater than 30 kg/m^2. It had been shown that 1% change in body weight predicts a 3% change in apnea-hypopnea index.

Neck Circumference. Men with neck circumference greater than 17" (43cm) and women with neck circumference greater than 16" (41cm) had been shown to be at significantly higher risk for OSA.

Being older. Prevalence of OSA is higher among elderly patients when compared with middle-aged persons.

Being of certain ethnicity. Prevalence of OSA is higher in African-Americans and Asians when compared with Caucasians.

Other risk factors include:

- Smoking
- Diabetes
- High blood pressure
- Being at risk for heart failure or stroke

What is it doing to people?

OSA posts significant risk to the patient's health due to constant disruption of sleep and lack of oxygen to vital organs.

Common signs and symptoms are:

- Daytime sleepiness or fatigue

- Dry mouth or sore throat when you wake up
- Headaches in the morning
- Trouble concentrating, forgetfulness, depression, or irritability
- Night sweats
- Restlessness during sleep
- Problems with sex
- Snoring
- Waking up suddenly and feeling like you're gasping or choking
- Trouble getting up in the mornings

Left untreated for a long time, OSA is associated with reduced quality of life, decreased cardiovascular health and increased healthcare utilization, motor vehicle accidents and mortality. The inability to breath during sleep causes hypertension, which eventually can lead to heart failure, and even "unexplained" nocturnal death. OSA had also been found to increase risk of stroke and all related deaths by two times. The frequent arousal from sleep results in sleep fragmentation and sleep deprivation. This can result in excessive daytime sleepiness, intellectual deterioration, personality changes, and behavioral disorders.

OSA had also been shown to be related to headache and chronic craniofacial pain. It was reported in a recent review article published in Sleep Medicine Reviews that 30-70% of OSA patients suffer from headaches. Although no relationship has been found between OSA and migraine in the general population, migraine in patients with OSA improves when OSA is treated. Temporal Mandibular Joint Disorder (TMD) is also found to be associated with OSA (28%).

How is it diagnosed?

Diagnosis of OSA is made by a physician who specializes in Sleep Medicine, using information collected from medical and family history, physical examination, and sleep study results. Nevertheless, the screening process usually starts with the family physician, family dentist, or even by the patients themselves.

STOP-BANG questionnaire is a quick but effective screening tool to identify those who are at high risk for OSA. It consists of 8 questions:

- **Snoring ?** Do you **Snore Loudly** (loud enough to be heard through closed doors or your bed-partner elbows you for snoring at night)?

- **Tired** ? Do you often feel **Tired, Fatigued, or Sleepy** during the daytime (such as falling asleep during driving or talking to someone)?
- **Observed** ? Has anyone **Observed you Stop Breathing or Choking/Gasping** during your sleep ?
- **Pressure** ? Do you have or are being treated for High Blood Pressure ?
- **Body Mass Index more than 35 kg/m^2?**
  BMI is calculated using the formula:
  Weight / Height^2
  [Weight (in kg) divided by square of height (in meter)]
- **Age older than 50 ?**
- **Neck size large ?** (Measured around Adams apple)
  For male, is your shirt collar 17 inches / 43cm or larger?
- For female, is your shirt collar 16 inches / 41cm or larger?
- **Gender = Male ?**

For the general population:

OSA - Low Risk : Yes to 0 - 2 questions

OSA - Intermediate Risk : Yes to 3 - 4 questions

OSA - High Risk : Yes to 5 - 8 questions

or Yes to 2 or more of 4 STOP questions + male gender

or Yes to 2 or more of 4 STOP questions + BMI > 35kg/m2

or Yes to 2 or more of 4 STOP questions + neck circumference 17 inches / 43cm in male or 16 inches / 41cm in female

Patients with intermediate to high OSA risk as identified by the STOP-BANG questionnaire should be referred to a sleep specialist for further investigation, usually require the use of a sleep study. Sleep studies are tests that measure how well a patient sleeps and the body responds to sleep problems. These tests can help the physician identify the presence of a sleep disorder and how severe it is.

Attended, in-laboratory polysomnography (poly-SOM-no-gram; also called a PSG) is considered the gold standard in the diagnosis of OSA. It is done at a sleep center or sleep lab, where the patient go to sleep as usual but with sensors attached to the scalp, face, chest, limbs, and a finger. A sleep technician will use the sensors to check on the patient throughout the night.

This study records brain activity, eye movements, heart rate, blood pressure, amount of oxygen in blood, and air movement through nose while breathing, snoring, and chest movements. The chest movements show if it takes an effort to breathe.

A sleep specialist will review the results of the PSG to determine presence and severity of OSA. The diagnosis of OSA is confirmed if the number of obstructive events per hour of sleep (apneas, hypopneas + respiratory event related arousals/hour of sleep; called respiratory disturbance index - RDI) on polysomnography is greater than 15 events/hour or greater than 5/hour in a patient who reports any of the following: unintentional sleep episodes during wakefulness; daytime sleepiness; unrefreshing sleep; fatigue; insomnia; waking up breath holding, gasping, or choking; or the bed partner describing loud snoring, breathing interruptions, or both during the patient's sleep. Obstructive sleep apnea severity is defined as mild for RDI 5 and < 15, moderate for RDI 15 and 30, and severe for RDI > 30/hr.

How is it Treated?

There are many possible treatment options:

1. **Weight Loss** (If needed): As mentioned, 1% change in BMI is associated with 3% change in severity of OSA. Losing even 10% of weight can make a significant difference.

2. **Avoid alcohol and sleeping pills:** Sedatives relaxes muscles, and make the airway more prone to collapse during sleep and hence increase the risk of OSA.

3. **Sleeping on your side:** Some patients may have mild OSA only when sleep on their back. This can be identified with a sleep study. For these patients, changing to sleeping on their sides may eliminate their OSA.

4. **CPAP Machine:** Continuous Positive Air Pressure (CPAP) machine is a device that forces constant and continuous air through the nose or mouth to create an air splint that keeps the upper airway open during sleep. In a Cochrane systemic review, CPAP showed significant improvements in objective and subjective

sleepiness, measures the quality of life, and cognitive function. Twenty-four hour systolic and diastolic blood pressure were also lower in patients treated with CPAP when compared with the control. Therefore, CPAP is currently the treatment of choice for patients with OSA. Nevertheless, CPAP is cumbersome to wear and compliance with therapy remains a difficult issue. It was found that 31% of patients never commenced therapy after initial diagnosis and CPAP titration. An additional 15% abandoned CPAP use after 10 months. Overall, it was found that only 54% of patients are able to tolerate the CPAP machine long term (after 64 months).

5. **Oral Appliance (OA):** Oral appliances are also called dental orthotics, tongue retaining devices, mandibular advancement appliances (MAA), mandibular advancement splints (MAS) or mandibular advancement devices (MAD). Oral appliances help to improve the potency of the airway through a combination of mechanisms, including: providing a stable and consistent, forward positioning of mandible, advancement of the tongue and possibly a change in the tongue muscle activity.

According to the guidelines of the Canadian Thoracic Society and the American Academy of Sleep Medicine (AASM), OAs in the adult population are recommended as a first-line therapy option for patients with primary snoring (without apnea) and for patients suffering from mild to moderate OSA who prefer an OA to CPAP therapy. Oral appliances are also an alternative therapy for patients with severe OSA who cannot tolerate CPAP, are inappropriate candidates for CPAP, or who have undergone failed CPAP treatment attempts.

The use of OA for an OSA patient should be prescribed by the physician who made the OSA diagnosis. An effective MAS is custom made for the patient using digital or physical impressions and models of patient's mouth and teeth. It is not a primarily prefabricated item that is trimmed, bent, relined, or otherwise modified. Therefore, OSA patients who are suitable are referred to a dentist for oral appliance therapy.

Although OA is less effective in reducing AHI in patients with moderate to severe OSA when compared to CPAP (CPAP AHI = 4.5; OA AHI = 11.1), the reported compliance was higher on OA (6.5hr/night vs. CPAP, 5.2hr/night). Overall, both appliance showed similar effectiveness in treating patients with OSA.

Children with OSA

Sleep apnea in infants was first identified in 1975 as sudden infant death syndrome and OSA. Today, OSA in children is recognized as the most severe form of the disease continuum of Sleep Disordered Breathing. American Academy of Pediatricians found that AHI of 1.5 events per hour or greater is abnormal for children, and 1-4% of children have OSA. Although both adult and children with OSA may have snoring, labored breathing during sleep, and high blood pressure, children with OSA can often be underweight and may not have daytime sleepiness. Instead, they could have attention-deficient/hyperactivity disorder. Left untreated, OSA has been shown to affect school performance and intellectual function, especially short term memory and concentration ability. Other sequelae include hypertension, cardiovascular failure, and frequent upper airway infections, as well as disturbances of growth and mood.

Similar to adult, the gold standard in diagnosis of OSA in children is in-laboratory, attended polysomnography sleep study. The first line of treatment for children with OSA is tonsillectomy and adenoidectomy (T&A), and it has been shown that removing both the tonsils and adenoids is more effective than either on its own. T & A had been shown to significantly improve obstructive symptoms in 80% of the cases; nevertheless, 13% of children who were successfully treated with T&A showed recurrence of symptoms when they reached adolescence.

For those children with OSA who have a constricted maxilla, an anterior open bite, and a long lower facial height, orthodontic treatment may be necessary, especially if they do not experience significant improvement in their dentofacial features and OSA symptoms even after removal of the adenoid and tonsils at an early age. **Rapid maxillary expansion (RME)** is an orthodontic treatment that widens the upper jaw through expansion forces appliance on the upper teeth. It is able to achieve widening of the upper jaw and the base of the nose, hence increasing the nasal passage and reducing the resistance to airflow. **Function mandibular advancement appliances (FMA)** change the posture of the mandible, holding it open and forward, and increase the potency of upper airway. These appliances are considered a moderately effective treatment for snoring and mild to moderate OSA in adult patients. In children, the appliance had been shown to induce differential growth and teeth movement between upper and lower jaws. It was found that treatment of OSA with an oral appliance (OA) in children with suitable malocclusions is an effective and well-tolerated method.

About the Author

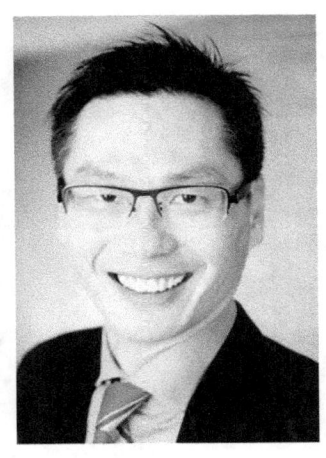

A first generation Canadian, Dr. Cheng Lun Wang spent his formative years in Toronto Canada. He received his formal education from Universities throughout Canada, including University of Toronto, University of Western Ontario, and University of Manitoba for his MSc. degree and certificate of Orthodontics specialty

Doctor Wang holds strongly to his inherited believe in family values and a sense of social responsibility, that every person should make a positive contribution to the community. Dr. Wang's professional career spans residency at The Hospital for Sick Children in Toronto, Resident Dentist at IWK Children's Hospital in Halifax, before settling down in private orthodontic practice in Vancouver, Canada.

Presently, Dr. Wang teaches clinical orthodontics at University of British Columbia, practice orthodontics in two private orthodontic clinics and more recently, started BC Head-Pain Institute in Vancouver, Canada. He shares his life with his wife and three children.